Title: **Low Glycemic Index diet Cookbook for beginners**

Subtitle: **Ultimate Guide to Healthy Eating for beginners on a Low Glycemic Index Diet**

By

Max Downs

Table of contents

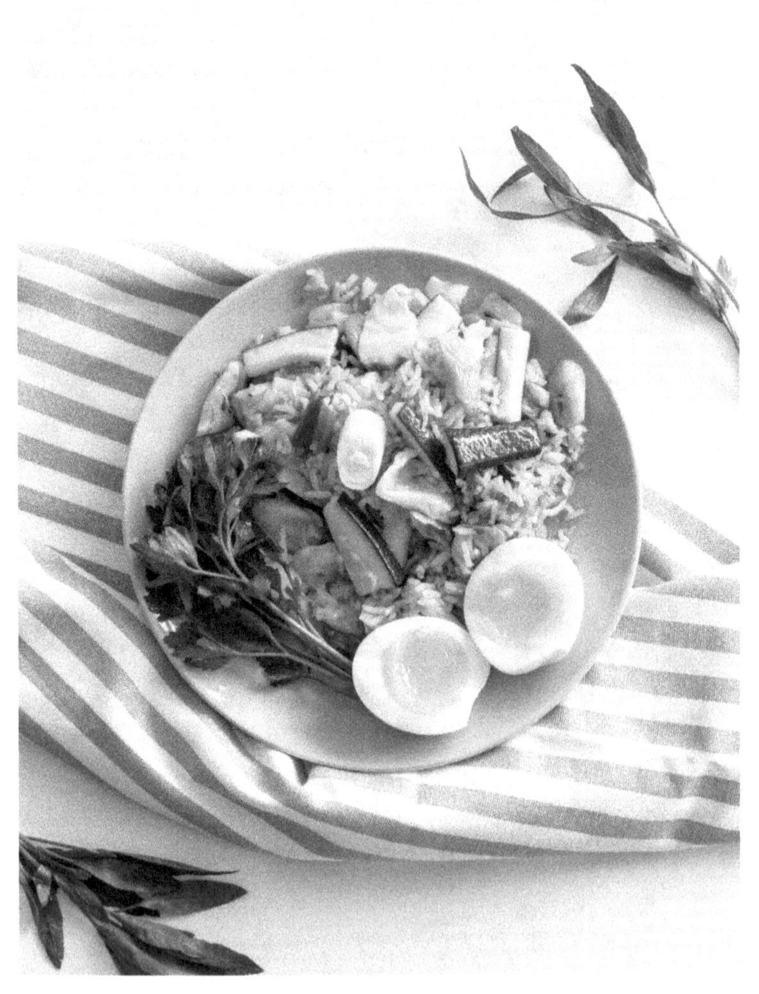

Introduction

Welcome to the culinary journey that promises not only delicious meals but also a path to improved health and vitality—the "Low Glycemic Index Diet Cookbook for Beginners."

In this cookbook, we embark on a transformative exploration into the realm of balanced and mindful eating. Designed specifically for beginners, this book serves as a compass, guiding you through the principles and practices of the low glycemic index (GI) diet.

Unlock the mysteries behind the glycemic index as we unravel the science, empowering you to make informed choices about the foods you consume. Discover how to utilise this knowledge to curate meals that stabilise blood sugar levels, enhance energy, and promote overall well-being.

Within these pages, you'll find a diverse array of recipes spanning breakfast, lunch, dinner, snacks, and even delectable desserts—each carefully crafted to not only tantalise your taste buds but also align with the principles of the low GI diet.

Join us on this flavorful expedition, where every meal becomes an opportunity to nourish your body, embrace vitality, and lay the foundation for a sustainable, health-conscious lifestyle. Whether you're taking your first steps into the world of low GI eating or seeking inspiration for culinary innovation, this cookbook serves as your trusted companion on the path to wholesome and delightful dining.

Understanding the concept and benefits of the low glycemic index diet.

The low glycemic index (GI) diet revolves around a fundamental principle: the impact of different foods on blood sugar levels. Understanding this concept involves delving into how carbohydrates affect our bodies after consumption.

Carbohydrates are the primary source of energy for the body, but not all carbs are created equal. The glycemic index is a scale that ranks foods based on how quickly they raise blood sugar levels after consumption. Foods with a high GI score cause a rapid spike in blood sugar, while those with a low GI score lead to a slower, more gradual increase.

By focusing on foods with a low GI, individuals can manage blood sugar levels more effectively. This approach offers several benefits, including:

1.**Stable Blood Sugar:** Low GI foods help maintain steady blood sugar levels, reducing the risk of sudden spikes and crashes, which can affect energy levels and hunger.

2.**Improved Satiety:** These foods tend to keep you fuller for longer periods, aiding in appetite control and potentially supporting weight management.

3.Better Diabetes Management: For individuals with diabetes, incorporating low GI foods into their diet can assist in better blood sugar control.

4.Enhanced Heart Health: Some research suggests that a low GI diet may contribute to better heart health by improving cholesterol levels and reducing the risk of heart disease.

Embracing the low GI diet involves choosing foods like whole grains, legumes, fruits, vegetables, and lean proteins that have a lower impact on blood sugar levels. This dietary approach not only fosters a more balanced way of eating but also promotes overall health and well-being.

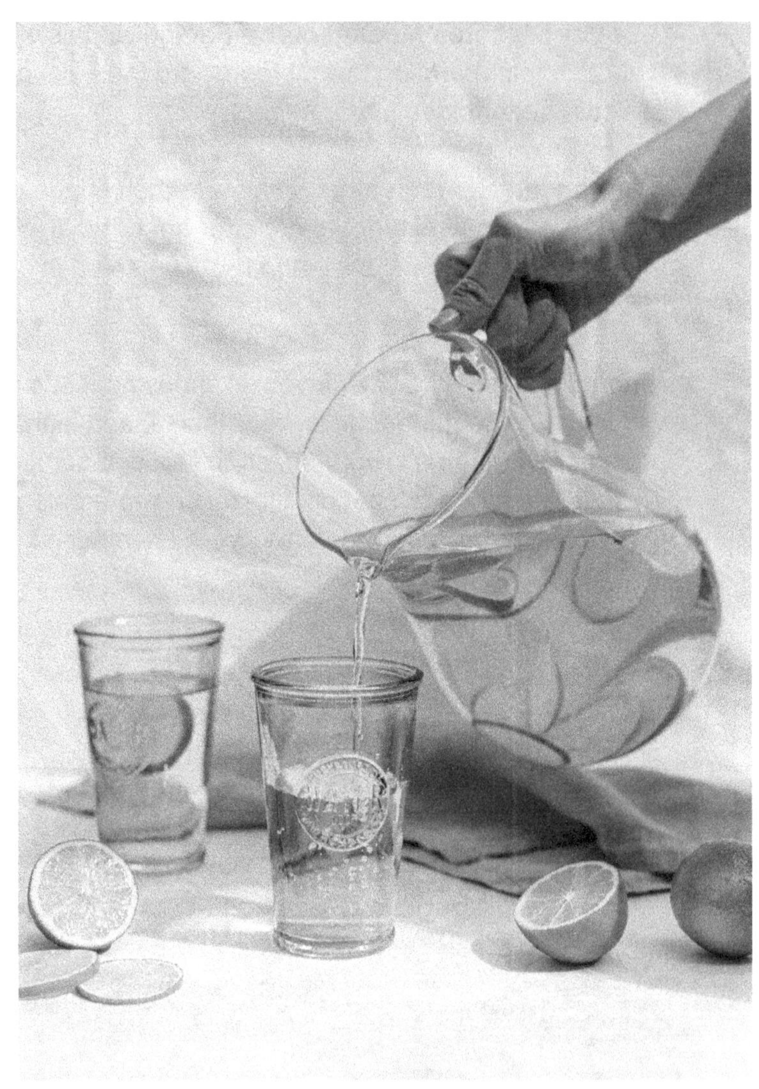

Chapter One

Understanding Glycemic Index

The Glycemic Index (GI) is a scale used to measure how different carbohydrate-containing foods affect blood sugar levels after consumption. This index ranks foods on a scale of 0 to 100 based on how quickly they cause blood sugar levels to rise.

Here's a breakdown of the Glycemic Index:

Low GI (55 or less): Foods with a low GI are digested and absorbed slowly, causing a gradual and modest rise in blood sugar levels. They provide sustained energy and help maintain stable blood sugar levels.

Medium GI (56-69): Foods in this range moderately raise blood sugar levels. They are absorbed at a moderate rate compared to high GI foods but still faster than low GI foods.

High GI (70 or more): These foods cause a rapid spike in blood sugar levels shortly after consumption. They are quickly digested and absorbed, resulting in a rapid increase in blood glucose.

Understanding the Glycemic Index assists in making informed dietary choices. By opting for foods with a lower GI, individuals can manage blood sugar levels more effectively, potentially reducing the risk of various health issues related to blood sugar fluctuations.

However, it's important to note that the GI of a food can be influenced by several factors, including ripeness, processing, cooking methods, and food combinations. As such, using the GI as a sole guide for meal planning may have limitations, and incorporating a variety of nutrient-rich, whole foods remains key for a balanced diet.

Delving deeper into the science behind the glycemic index and its impact on health.

The Glycemic Index (GI) has a profound impact on our health, serving as a valuable tool in understanding how different foods affect our bodies' glucose levels and overall well-being.

The science behind the Glycemic Index delves into the intricate mechanisms of carbohydrate metabolism. When we consume carbohydrates, our digestive system breaks them down into glucose, which enters the bloodstream, affecting blood sugar levels. Foods with a higher GI cause a rapid increase in blood sugar, while those with a lower GI result in a more gradual and sustained rise.

1.Energy Regulation: Foods with a lower GI provide a steady and sustained release of energy, promoting consistent energy levels throughout the day. In contrast, high-GI foods can lead to energy spikes followed by crashes.

2.Blood Sugar Management: For individuals with diabetes or those at risk of insulin resistance, understanding and incorporating lower GI foods into the diet can assist in managing blood sugar levels more effectively.

3.Weight Management: Lower-GI foods tend to keep you feeling fuller for longer periods, potentially aiding in appetite control and weight management by reducing overall calorie intake.

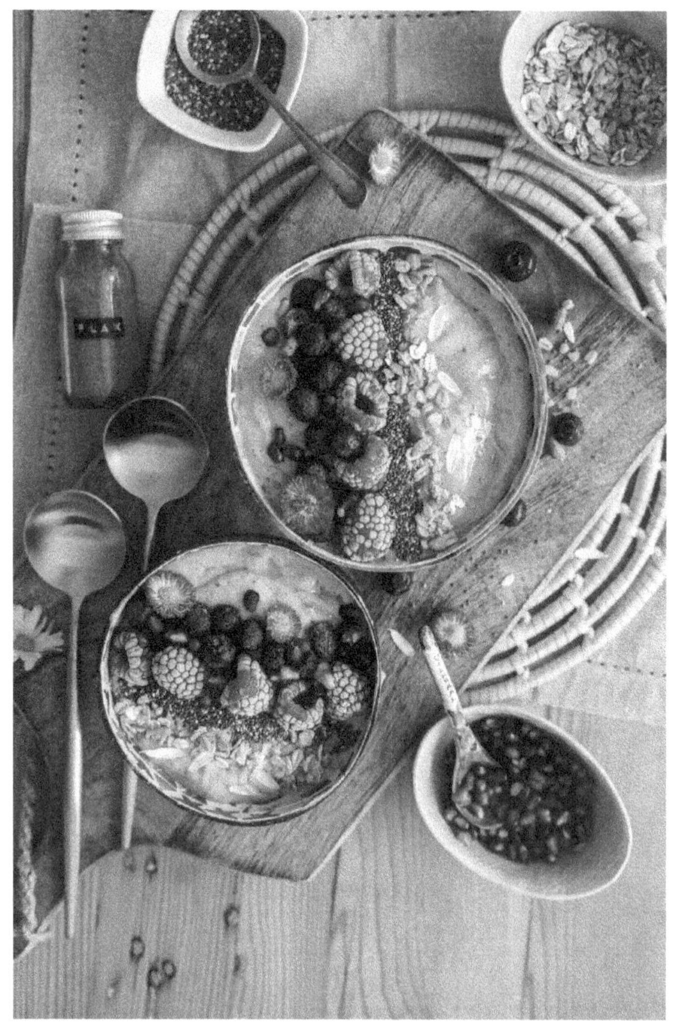

4.Heart Health: Some research suggests that diets emphasising lower-GI foods may contribute to better heart health by improving cholesterol levels and reducing the risk of heart disease.

However, it's important to approach the Glycemic Index within the broader context of a balanced diet. Other factors, such as portion sizes, overall nutritional content, and individual metabolic differences, also play crucial roles in maintaining good health.

By understanding the science behind the Glycemic Index and its impact on health, individuals can make informed dietary choices to promote stable blood sugar levels, sustained energy, and overall well-being.

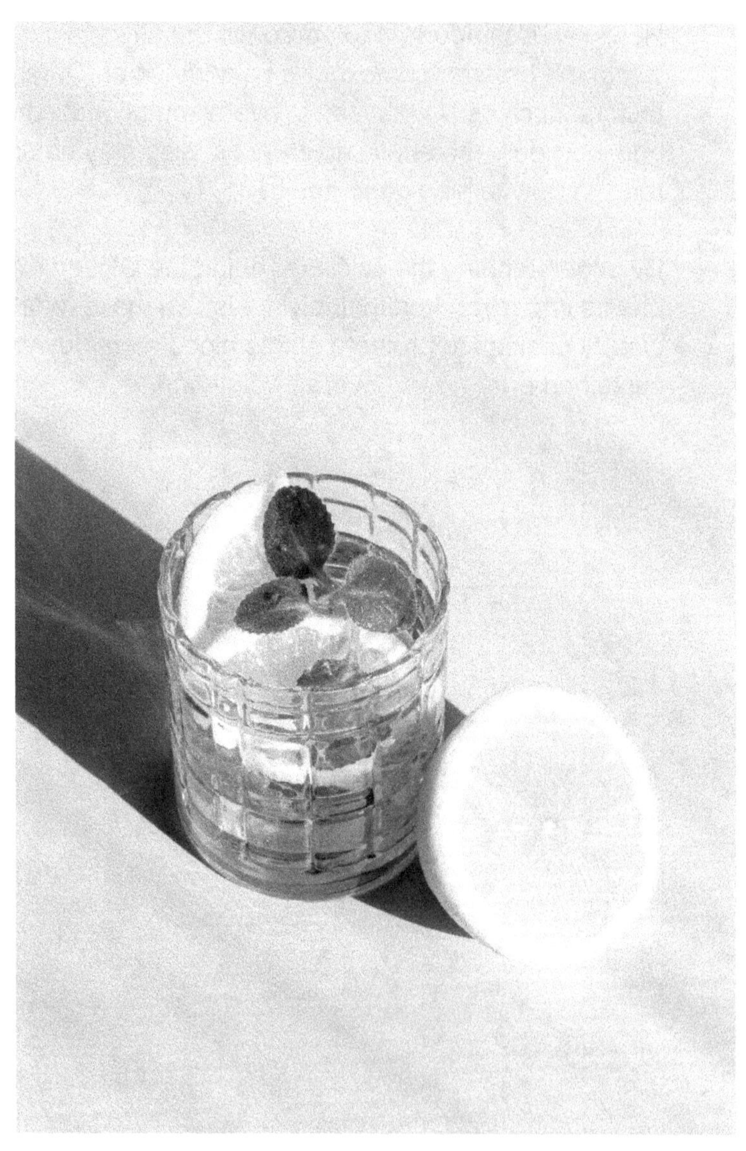

Chapter Two

Essential Ingredients and Pantry Staples

Stocking your pantry with essential ingredients for a low glycemic index (GI) diet sets the stage for creating wholesome, balanced meals. Here's a guide to essential pantry staples:

1.Whole Grains: Opt for whole grains like quinoa, brown rice, barley, oats, and whole wheat pasta. These are rich in fibre and have a lower impact on blood sugar compared to refined grains.

2.Legumes and Pulses: Include a variety of beans, lentils, and chickpeas. They're excellent sources of protein, fibre, and complex carbohydrates, contributing to a low GI diet.

3.Healthy Fats: Choose sources of healthy fats such as extra virgin olive oil, avocados, nuts (almonds, walnuts), and seeds (chia, flaxseeds). These fats help regulate blood sugar levels and provide essential nutrients.

4.Fresh Produce: Load up on colourful vegetables and fruits. Aim for a diverse range, including leafy greens, broccoli, tomatoes, berries, citrus fruits, and others with lower glycemic loads.

5.Lean Proteins: Incorporate lean protein sources like skinless poultry, fish, tofu, tempeh, and eggs. Protein helps slow down the digestion of carbohydrates, reducing their glycemic impact.

6.Dairy or Dairy Alternatives: Choose low-fat dairy products or dairy alternatives like unsweetened almond milk, soy milk, or Greek yoghurt (unsweetened) to add calcium and protein to your diet.

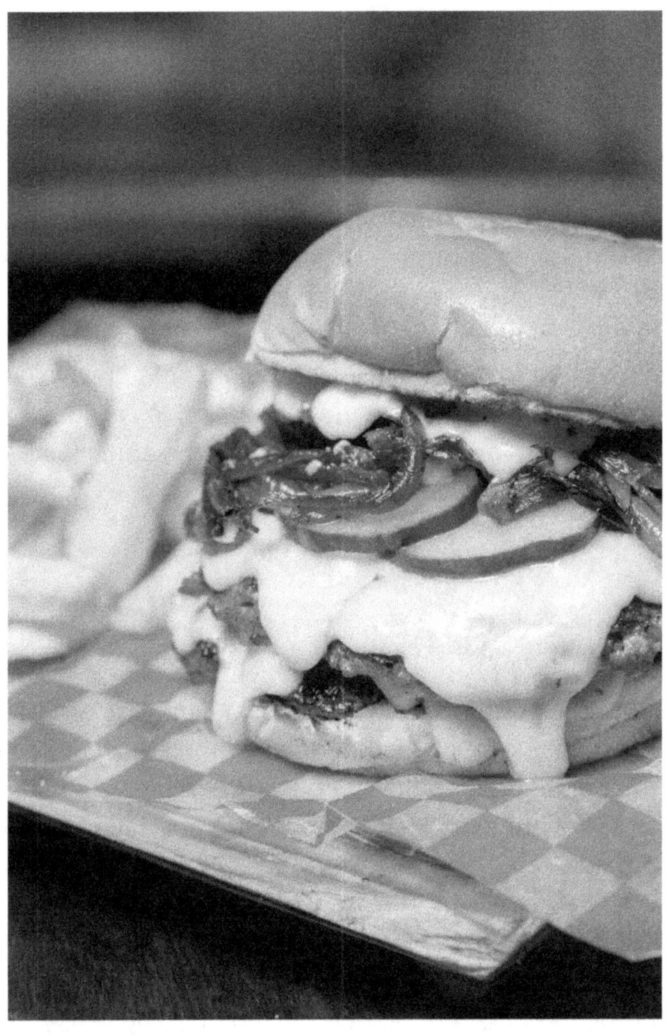

7.Herbs, Spices, and Flavour Enhancers: Stock up on herbs, spices, and seasonings to add flavour without relying on high-GI sauces or condiments. Think garlic, turmeric, cinnamon, cumin, paprika, etc.

8.Low GI Sweeteners: Use sweeteners like stevia, erythritol, or monk fruit extract sparingly to add sweetness without spiking blood sugar levels.

9.Whole Food Snacks: Keep snacks on hand that are low in added sugars and high in nutrients, such as unsalted nuts, seeds, or air-popped popcorn.

By having these essential ingredients readily available in your pantry, you'll have the foundation to create nourishing, low GI meals that support stable blood sugar levels and overall health.

A comprehensive guide to stocking your kitchen for successful low GI cooking.

Stocking your kitchen for successful low glycemic index (GI) cooking involves thoughtful planning and selecting the right ingredients. Here's a comprehensive guide to ensure your kitchen is equipped for delicious low GI meals:

1.Whole Grains: Fill your pantry with whole grains like quinoa, brown rice, bulgur, barley, oats, and whole wheat products. These provide fibre and nutrients while maintaining a lower GI.

2.Legumes and Pulses: Include a variety of beans such as black beans, kidney beans, lentils, and chickpeas.

They're rich in protein, fibre, and complex carbs, ideal for low GI meals.

3.Fresh Produce: Load up on a rainbow of vegetables and fruits. Opt for leafy greens, broccoli, carrots, tomatoes, bell peppers, berries, apples, and citrus fruits. These offer nutrients and fibre with lower glycemic loads.

4.Lean Proteins: Stock up on lean protein sources like skinless poultry, fish, tofu, tempeh, eggs, and low-fat dairy products. Protein helps stabilise blood sugar levels when combined with low GI carbohydrates.

5.Healthy Fats: Choose sources of healthy fats such as extra virgin olive oil, avocados, nuts (almonds, walnuts), and seeds (chia, flaxseeds). They contribute to satiety and assist in blood sugar regulation.

6.Dairy or Dairy Alternatives: Include low-fat dairy products or dairy alternatives like unsweetened almond milk, soy milk, or Greek yoghurt (unsweetened) for calcium and protein.

7.Herbs, Spices, and Flavour Enhancers: Build a collection of herbs, spices, and seasonings to enhance flavour without relying on high-GI sauces or condiments. Garlic, turmeric, cinnamon, cumin, and paprika are great choices.

8.Low GI Sweeteners: Have low GI sweeteners like stevia, erythritol, or monk fruit extract on hand for occasional sweetening needs without impacting blood sugar levels significantly.

9.Whole Food Snacks: Keep whole food snacks available, such as unsalted nuts, seeds, air-popped popcorn, or veggie sticks. They make for nutritious low-GI snack options.

10.Cooking Essentials: Ensure your kitchen is stocked with essential cooking tools, including a variety of pots and pans, a blender, food processor, sharp knives, and measuring utensils to facilitate meal preparation.

By maintaining a well-stocked kitchen with these low GI ingredients and cooking essentials, you'll have the foundation to create flavorful, nutrient-rich meals that support stable blood sugar levels and overall health.

Chapter Three

Building Balanced Meals

Building balanced meals within a low glycemic index (GI) framework is key to optimising nutrition and maintaining stable blood sugar levels. Here's a guide to constructing balanced meals:

1.Incorporate Low GI Carbohydrates: Choose whole grains like quinoa, brown rice, barley, or whole wheat products as the base of your meal. These provide sustained energy without causing rapid blood sugar spikes.

2.Add Lean Proteins: Include lean protein sources such as chicken, turkey, fish, tofu, tempeh, eggs, or legumes like lentils and beans. Protein helps regulate blood sugar levels and promotes satiety.

3.Load Up on Vegetables: Fill half of your plate with a colourful array of non-starchy vegetables like leafy greens, broccoli, bell peppers, carrots, and tomatoes. These provide essential vitamins, minerals, and fibre with minimal impact on blood sugar.

4.Incorporate Healthy Fats: Include sources of healthy fats like avocado, nuts, seeds, and olive oil in moderation. Fats contribute to satiety and slow down the digestion of carbohydrates, aiding in blood sugar regulation.

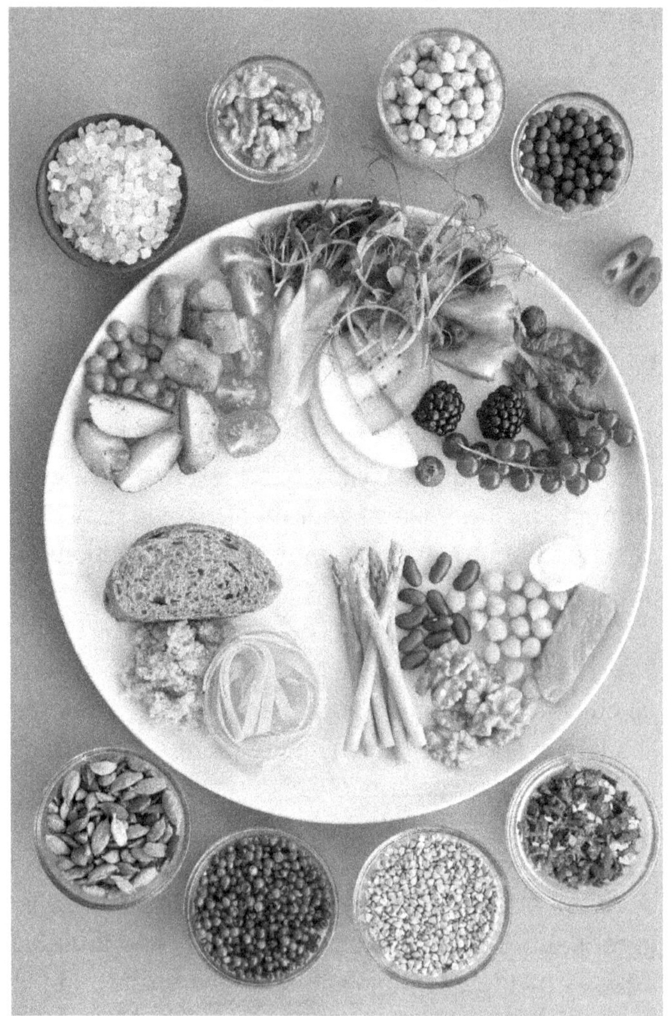

5.Mindful Portion Control: Pay attention to portion sizes to ensure a balanced intake of nutrients. Aim for a palm-sized portion of protein, a quarter plate of whole grains, and the remaining half plate filled with non-starchy vegetables.

6.Focus on Fibre: Include foods high in fibre, such as legumes, vegetables, fruits, and whole grains. Fibre slows down digestion, leading to a more gradual release of glucose into the bloodstream.

7.Hydration: Don't forget about hydration. Water is essential for overall health and can aid in digestion and maintaining stable blood sugar levels.

8.Balanced Snacking: If snacking, choose low GI options such as a handful of nuts, Greek yoghurt, or raw vegetables with hummus to keep blood sugar levels steady between meals.

9.Variety is Key: Aim for a diverse range of foods to ensure a wide spectrum of nutrients and flavours in your meals.

By creating meals that balance low GI carbohydrates, lean proteins, healthy fats, fibre-rich vegetables, and mindful portion sizes, you can enjoy well-rounded and satisfying meals while supporting stable blood sugar levels and overall health.

Certainly! Here are some tips and strategies for crafting well-rounded, low glycemic index (GI) meals:

1.**Focus on Whole Foods:** Emphasise whole, unprocessed foods such as whole grains, fresh fruits, vegetables, lean proteins, and healthy fats. These tend to have lower GI values compared to processed alternatives.

2.**Combine Foods Wisely:** Pair higher GI foods with low GI counterparts to balance the overall meal's glycemic impact. For instance, combine brown rice (low GI) with grilled chicken (protein) and a variety of colourful veggies for a balanced plate.

3.**Prioritize Fibre:** Incorporate high-fibre foods like legumes, beans, lentils, whole grains, and fibrous vegetables. Fibre slows down digestion, helping to stabilise blood sugar levels.

4.**Choose Low GI Carbs:** Opt for low GI carbohydrates such as quinoa, barley, bulgur, and steel-cut oats over high GI options like white rice or refined grains.

5.**Include Lean Proteins:** Incorporate lean protein sources like fish, poultry, tofu, tempeh, eggs, or legumes in each meal. Protein slows the digestion of carbohydrates, reducing their glycemic impact.

6.Healthy Fats in Moderation: Include sources of healthy fats like avocados, nuts, seeds, and olive oil. These fats aid in satiety and can help regulate blood sugar levels.

7.Experiment with Cooking Methods: Experiment with cooking methods like steaming, roasting, grilling, or sautéing with minimal oil to retain nutrients and flavours without adding unnecessary fats or sugars.

8.Add Flavor with Herbs and Spices: Use herbs, spices, and citrus juices to enhance flavour without relying on high-GI sauces or seasonings.

9.Mindful Portion Control: Be mindful of portion sizes. While healthy, even low GI foods can impact blood sugar if consumed excessively. Stick to appropriate serving sizes.

10.Meal Planning and Prepping: Plan your meals in advance to ensure a good balance of nutrients. Consider batch cooking or meal prepping to have low GI options readily available.

11.Stay Hydrated: Drink plenty of water throughout the day. Staying hydrated can support overall health and may help manage cravings.

By applying these tips and strategies, you can create satisfying, well-rounded meals that prioritise low GI foods, promoting stable blood sugar levels and supporting your overall health goals.

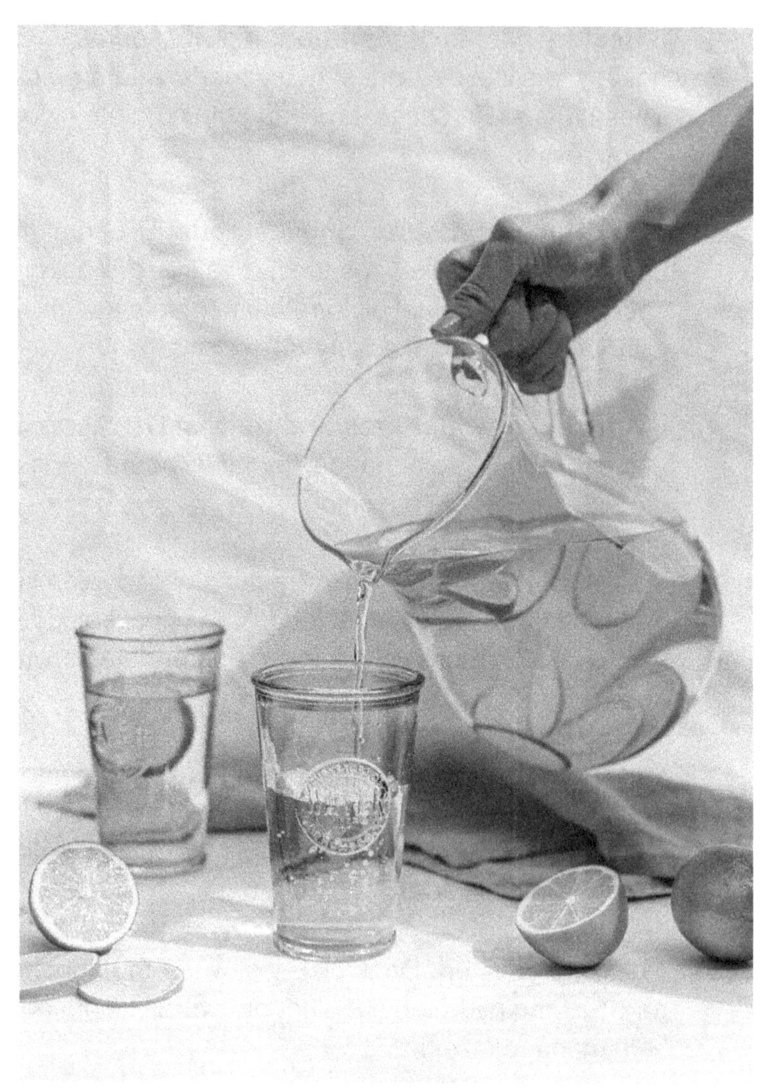

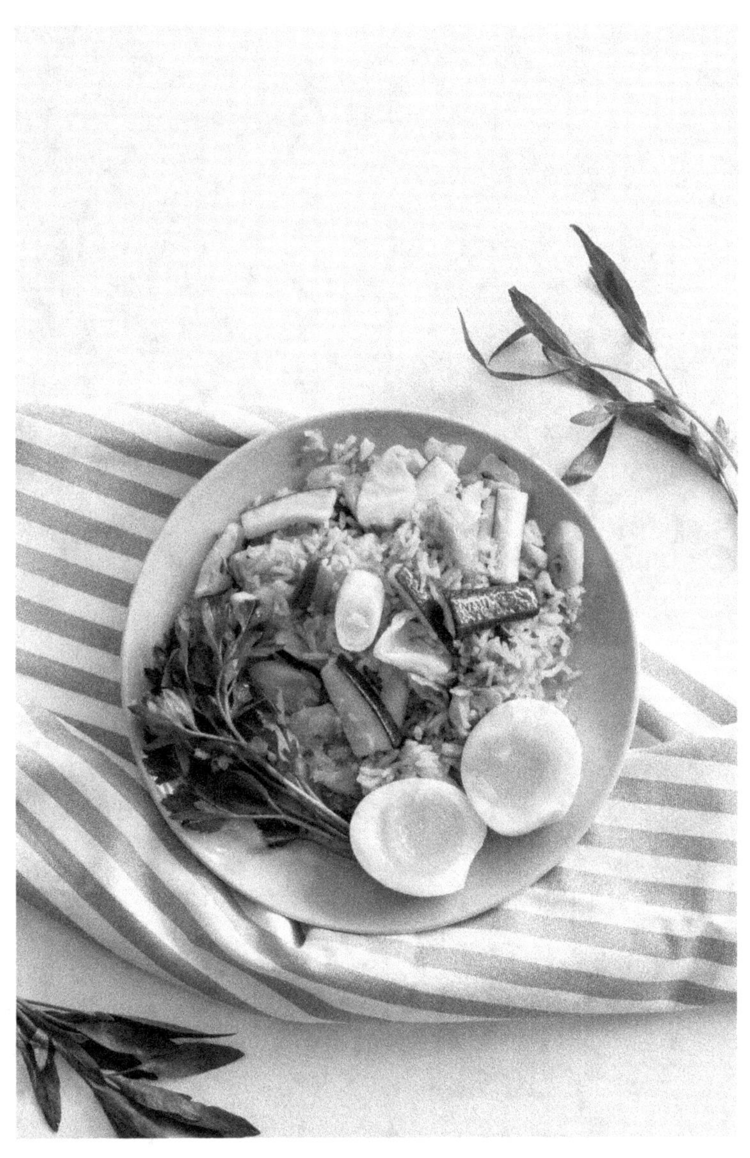

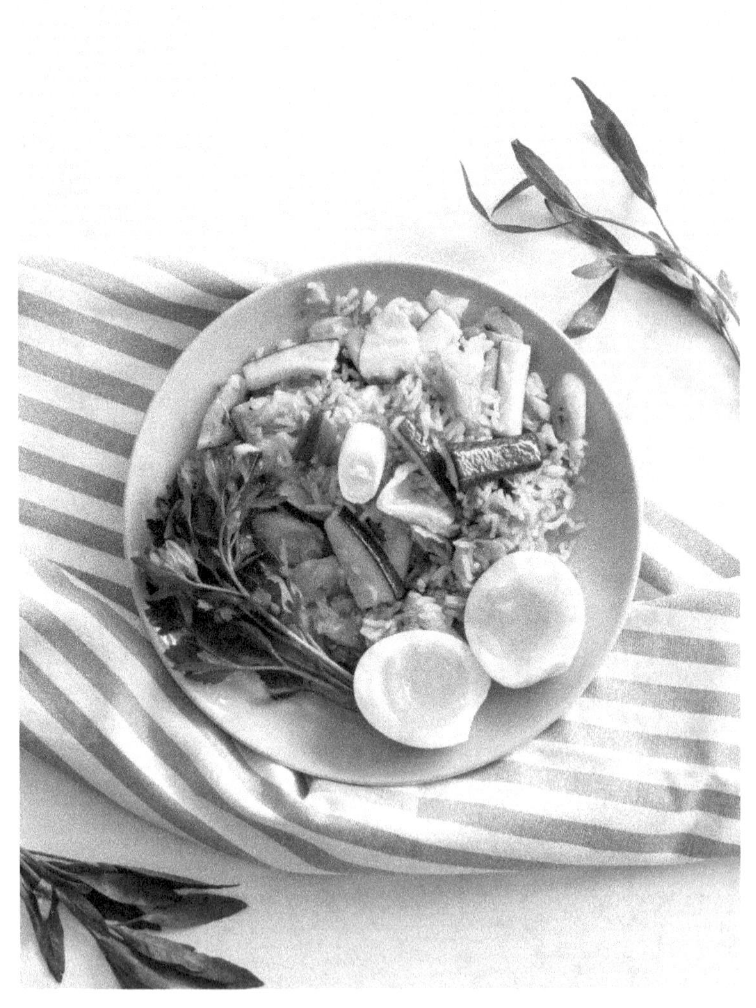

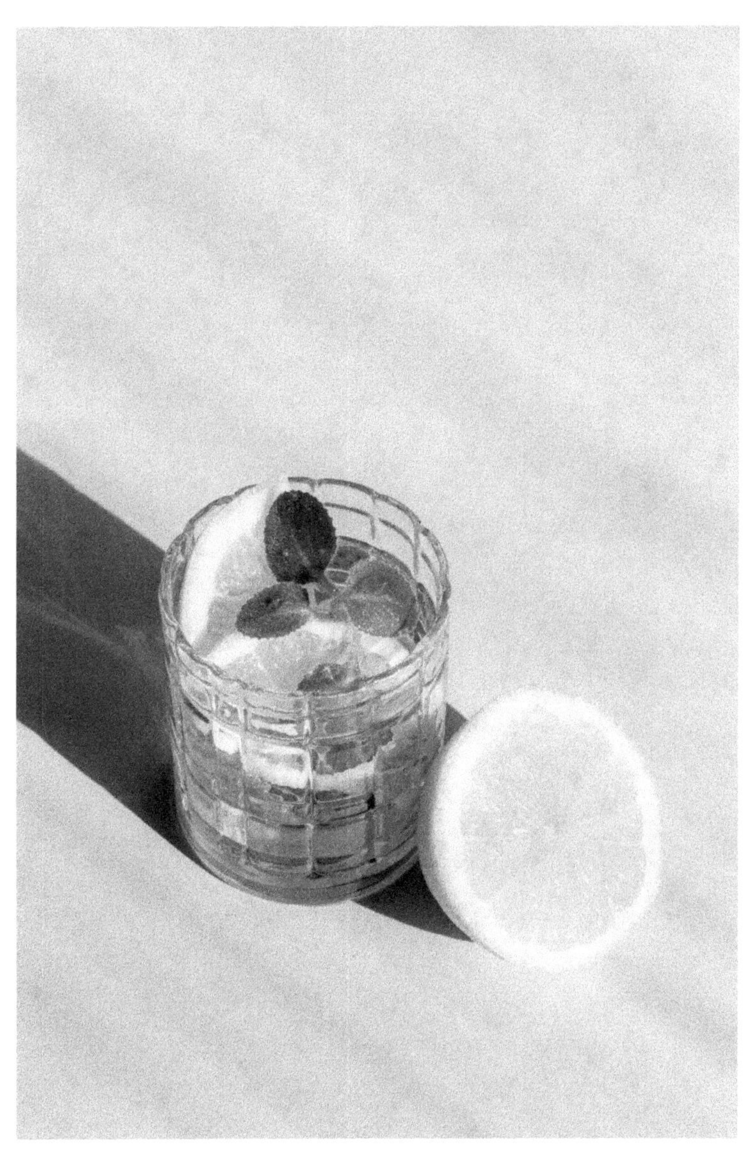

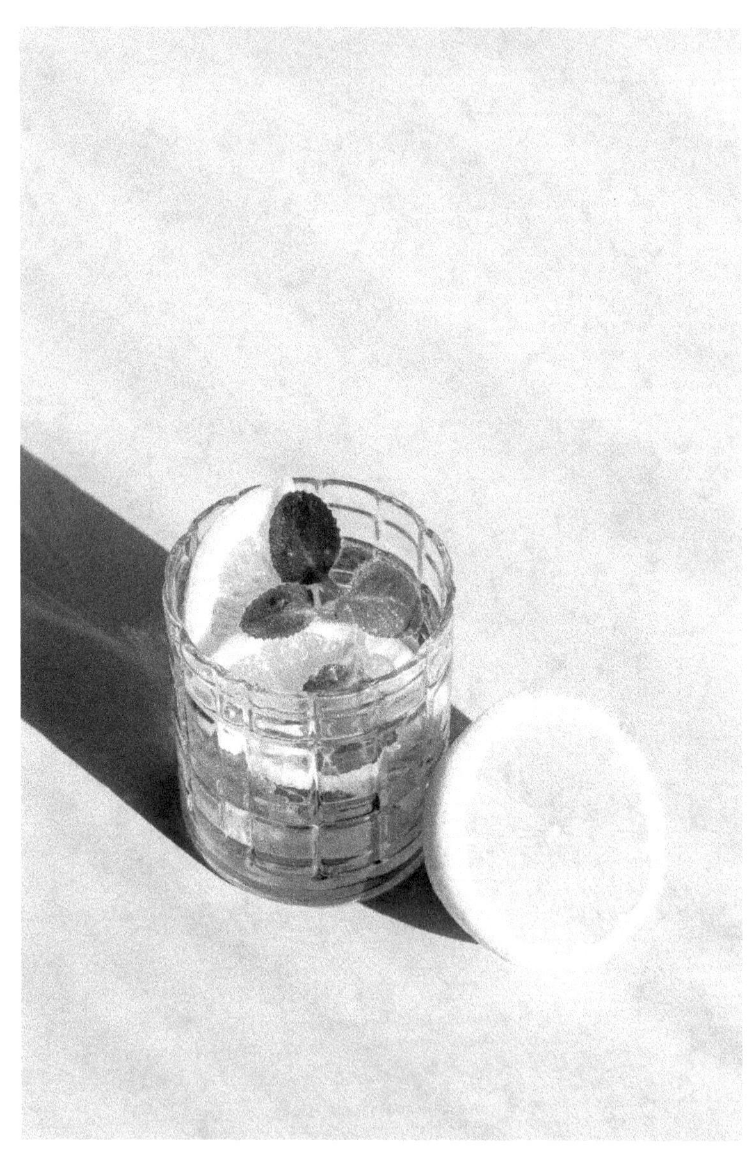

Chapter Four

Breakfast Boosts

Certainly! Here are some breakfast ideas that serve as excellent boosts for a low glycemic index (GI) diet:

1.Overnight Oats: Prepare oats with almond milk, chia seeds, and a dash of cinnamon. Top with fresh berries, nuts, or a dollop of Greek yoghurt for added protein and flavour.

2.Vegetable Omelette: Whip up an omelette with veggies like spinach, bell peppers, onions, and tomatoes. Pair it with whole grain toast or a side of avocado for healthy fats.

3.Greek Yogurt Parfait: Layer Greek yoghourt with low GI fruits like berries or sliced apples. Add a sprinkle of nuts or seeds for crunch and extra nutrients.

4.Quinoa Breakfast Bowl: Cook quinoa and mix it with coconut milk, nuts, and diced fruits like mango or kiwi. Drizzle with honey or a touch of vanilla extract for sweetness.

5.Chia Seed Pudding: Combine chia seeds with unsweetened almond milk, vanilla extract, and a touch of honey or stevia. Let it sit overnight and top with nuts or fruits in the morning.

6.Whole Grain Toast with Nut Butter: Spread almond or peanut butter on whole grain toast. Add sliced bananas or strawberries for a tasty, low GI option.

7.Egg and Veggie Muffin Cups: Bake eggs with chopped vegetables in muffin cups for a portable, protein-packed breakfast. Pair with a small serving of low GI fruit.

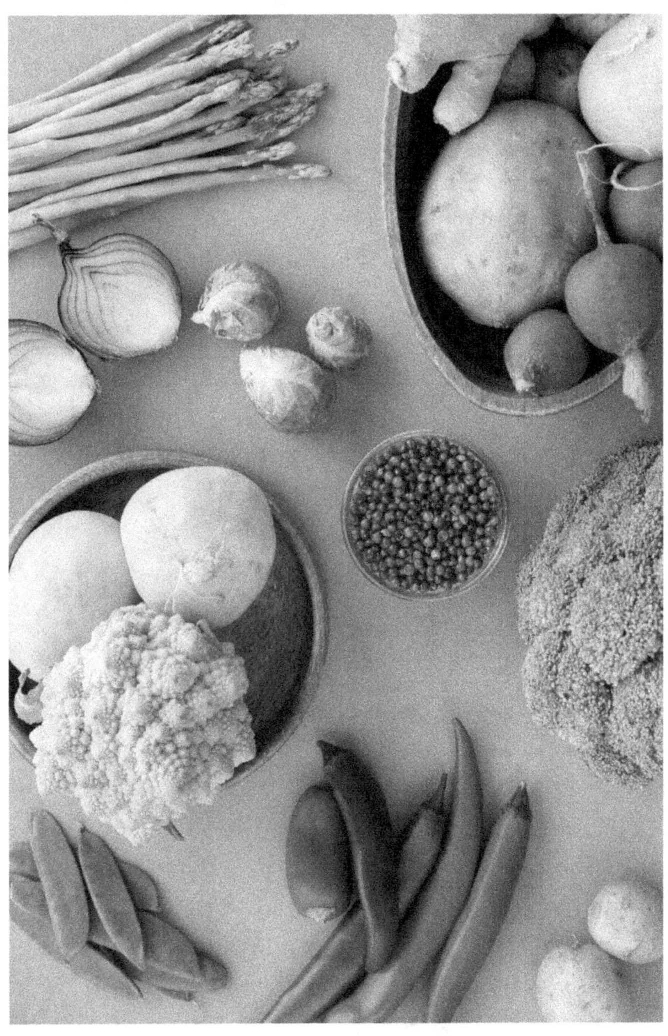

8.Savory Breakfast Burrito: Fill a whole grain wrap with scrambled eggs, black beans, diced tomatoes, and avocado. Serve with a side of salsa for added flavour.

9.Buckwheat Pancakes: Make pancakes using buckwheat flour and top with fresh fruit or a light drizzle of pure maple syrup.

10.Smoothie Bowl: Blend low GI fruits like berries or cherries with spinach, Greek yoghurt, and a splash of almond milk. Top with nuts, seeds, or granola for crunch.

These breakfast ideas are not only delicious but also incorporate low GI ingredients to help you start your day on the right nutritional foot, keeping your blood sugar levels stable and providing sustained energy.

Recipes and ideas for energising and low glycemic breakfast options.

Absolutely! Here are a few energising and low glycemic breakfast recipes:

Quinoa Breakfast Porridge
Ingredients:
1 cup cooked quinoa
1 cup almond milk (or any preferred milk)
1 tablespoon maple syrup or honey (optional)
½ teaspoon cinnamon
Fresh berries (such as blueberries or strawberries)
Chopped nuts (almonds, walnuts)
Unsweetened shredded coconut (optional)

Instructions:

1.In a saucepan, combine cooked quinoa, almond milk, maple syrup or honey (if using), and cinnamon.
2.Heat over medium-low heat, stirring occasionally, until warmed through and creamy.
3.Serve in bowls and top with fresh berries, chopped nuts, and shredded coconut if desired.

Egg and Spinach Breakfast Wrap
Ingredients:
2 large eggs
1 cup fresh spinach leaves
1 whole grain or low carb tortilla
Salt and pepper to taste
Sliced avocado (optional)
Salsa or hot sauce (optional)

Instructions:
1.In a non-stick skillet, sauté fresh spinach until wilted.
2.In the same skillet, scramble eggs with salt and pepper.
3.Warm the tortilla and lay it flat.
4.Place the scrambled eggs and sautéed spinach on the tortilla.
5.Add sliced avocado if desired and roll the tortilla into a wrap.
6.Serve with salsa or hot sauce if preferred.

Berry and Chia Seed Smoothie

Ingredients:
1 cup mixed berries (such as strawberries, raspberries, and blueberries)
1 tablespoon chia seeds

½ cup Greek yoghourt
1 cup unsweetened almond milk (or any preferred milk)
Honey or maple syrup (optional for sweetness)

Instructions:
1.Blend mixed berries, chia seeds, Greek yoghurt, and almond milk until smooth.
2.Add honey or maple syrup for sweetness if desired.
3.Pour into a glass and enjoy this nutritious and refreshing smoothie.
These recipes are not only energising but also incorporate low GI ingredients to help stabilise blood sugar levels and provide sustained energy throughout the morning. Feel free to customise these recipes based on personal preferences!

Chapter Five

Lunchtime Delights

Certainly! Here are a few lunchtime delights that are both satisfying and adhere to a low glycemic index (GI) diet:

Quinoa and Roasted Vegetable Salad

Ingredients:

1 cup cooked quinoa
Assorted roasted vegetables (bell peppers, zucchini, cherry tomatoes)
Mixed greens (spinach, arugula)
Feta cheese or goat cheese (optional)
Balsamic vinaigrette dressing

Instructions:
1.Toss cooked quinoa with roasted vegetables and mixed greens.
2.Crumble feta or goat cheese on top (if using).
3.Drizzle with balsamic vinaigrette dressing and toss gently before serving.

Grilled Chicken and Avocado Wrap

Ingredients:

Grilled chicken breast strips

Sliced avocado
Shredded lettuce
Whole grain wrap or tortilla
Greek yoghourt-based dressing or hummus

Instructions:
1.Lay out the whole grain wrap and spread Greek yoghourt-based dressing or hummus.
2. Layer grilled chicken, sliced avocado, and shredded lettuce.
3.Roll the wrap tightly, slice in half, and serve.

Lentil Soup with Greens

Ingredients:
1 cup cooked lentils
Chopped kale or spinach
Vegetable or chicken broth
Diced onions, carrots, and celery
Garlic, salt, pepper, and herbs for seasoning

Instructions:
1.In a pot, sauté onions, carrots, and celery until soft.
2.Add cooked lentils, chopped greens, and broth to the pot.
3.Season with garlic, salt, pepper, and herbs.
4.Simmer until the flavours meld together, and the greens are tender.

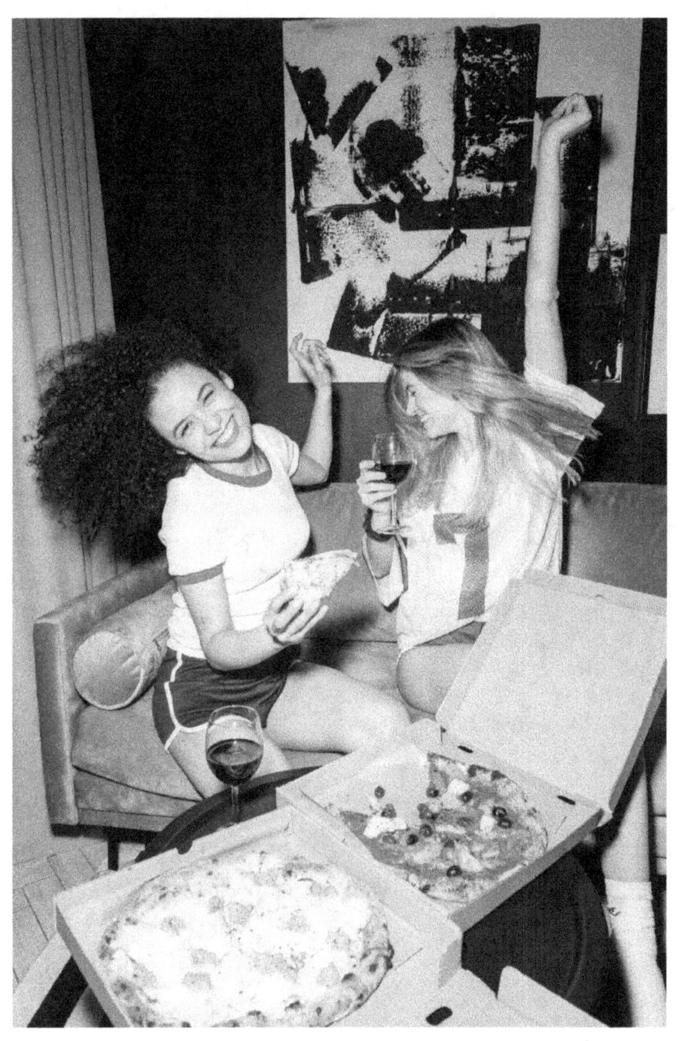

Tuna and White Bean Salad

Ingredients:

Canned tuna in water, drained
White beans (cannellini or navy beans)
Chopped red onions and celery
Chopped parsley
Lemon juice, olive oil, salt, and pepper for dressing

Instructions:
1.Mix canned tuna, white beans, red onions, celery, and chopped parsley in a bowl.
2.Dress with lemon juice, olive oil, salt, and pepper.
3.Serve over a bed of mixed greens or enjoy as a sandwich filling.
These lunch options are not only flavorful and satisfying but also incorporate low GI ingredients to help maintain stable blood sugar levels throughout the day. Adjust the recipes to suit personal tastes and dietary preferences!

Nutritious and satisfying lunch recipes suited for a low GI lifestyle

Absolutely! Here are some nutritious and satisfying lunch recipes suitable for a low glycemic index (GI) lifestyle:

Mediterranean Chickpea Salad

Ingredients:

1 can chickpeas (drained and rinsed)
Diced cucumber and tomatoes
Chopped red onion and bell peppers

Chopped fresh parsley and mint
Feta cheese (optional)
Olive oil, lemon juice, salt, and pepper for dressing

Instructions:
1.Combine chickpeas, diced vegetables, chopped herbs, and feta cheese (if using) in a bowl.
2.Drizzle with olive oil and lemon juice, season with salt and pepper, and toss gently before serving.

Grilled Veggie and Chicken Quinoa Bowl

Ingredients:

Grilled chicken breast strips
Assorted grilled vegetables (zucchini, eggplant, bell peppers)
Cooked quinoa
Baby spinach or arugula
Balsamic vinaigrette or tahini dressing

Instructions:
1.Arrange cooked quinoa, grilled chicken, grilled vegetables, and greens in a bowl.
2.Drizzle with balsamic vinaigrette or tahini dressing for added flavour.

Salmon and Avocado Salad

Ingredients:

Grilled or baked salmon fillet
Sliced avocado
Mixed greens (spinach, arugula)
Cherry tomatoes
Toasted pumpkin seeds or almonds
Lemon-tahini dressing

Instructions:
1.Arrange mixed greens, cherry tomatoes, sliced avocado, and salmon on a plate.
2.Sprinkle with toasted pumpkin seeds or almonds and drizzle with lemon-tahini dressing before serving.

Turkey and Vegetable Lettuce Wraps

Ingredients:

Ground turkey or chicken
Finely chopped mixed vegetables (carrots, bell peppers, mushrooms)
Lettuce leaves for wrapping
Hoisin sauce or low-sodium soy sauce
Sesame oil, garlic, ginger (for flavour)

Instructions:
1.Stir-fry ground turkey and chopped vegetables with garlic and ginger.
2.Season with hoisin sauce or low-sodium soy sauce and sesame oil.
3.Serve the mixture in lettuce leaves for a delicious wrap.

These recipes offer a blend of flavours, nutrients, and low GI ingredients to create satisfying lunches that help stabilise blood sugar levels while keeping you energised throughout the day. Adjust seasonings and ingredients according to personal preferences!

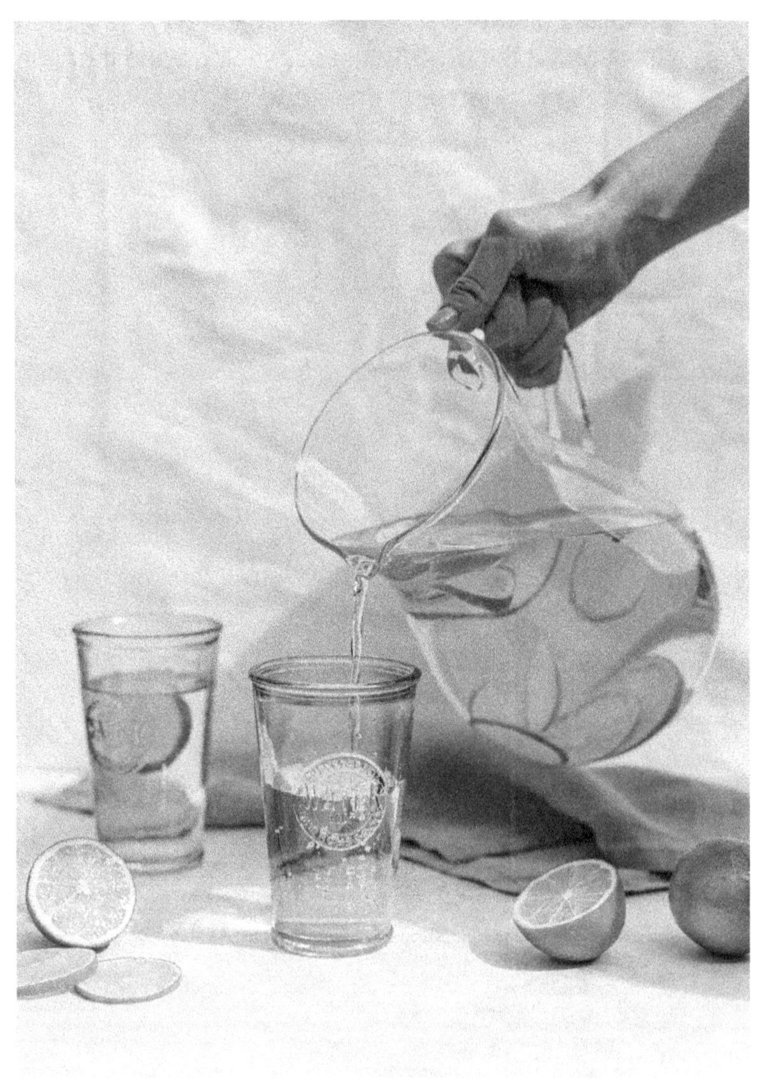

Chapter Six

Dinner Creations

Absolutely! Here are some flavorful and nutritious dinner creations aligned with a low glycemic index (GI) diet:

Baked Lemon Herb Chicken with Roasted Vegetables

Ingredients:

Chicken breasts or thighs
Lemon juice, garlic, olive oil, herbs (rosemary, thyme)
Assorted vegetables (bell peppers, broccoli, carrots)
Salt and pepper

Instructions:
1.Marinate chicken in lemon juice, garlic, olive oil, and herbs for at least 30 minutes.
2.Place the chicken in a baking dish and surround it with assorted vegetables.
3.Drizzle olive oil over the vegetables, season with salt and pepper, and bake until the chicken is cooked through and the veggies are tender.

Cauliflower and Chickpea Curry

Ingredients:

Cauliflower florets
Cooked chickpeas
Onion, garlic, ginger
Curry spices (turmeric, cumin, coriander)
Coconut milk or tomato-based sauce
Spinach or kale

Instructions:
1.Sauté onions, garlic, and ginger in a pan.
2.Add cauliflower, cooked chickpeas, and curry spices.
Cook until fragrant.
3.Pour in coconut milk or tomato-based sauce and
simmer until the cauliflower is tender.
4.Add spinach or kale at the end and cook until wilted

Salmon with Quinoa and Steamed Greens

Ingredients:

Salmon fillets
Cooked quinoa
Assorted steamed greens (spinach, kale, Swiss chard)
Lemon zest, olive oil, herbs (optional)

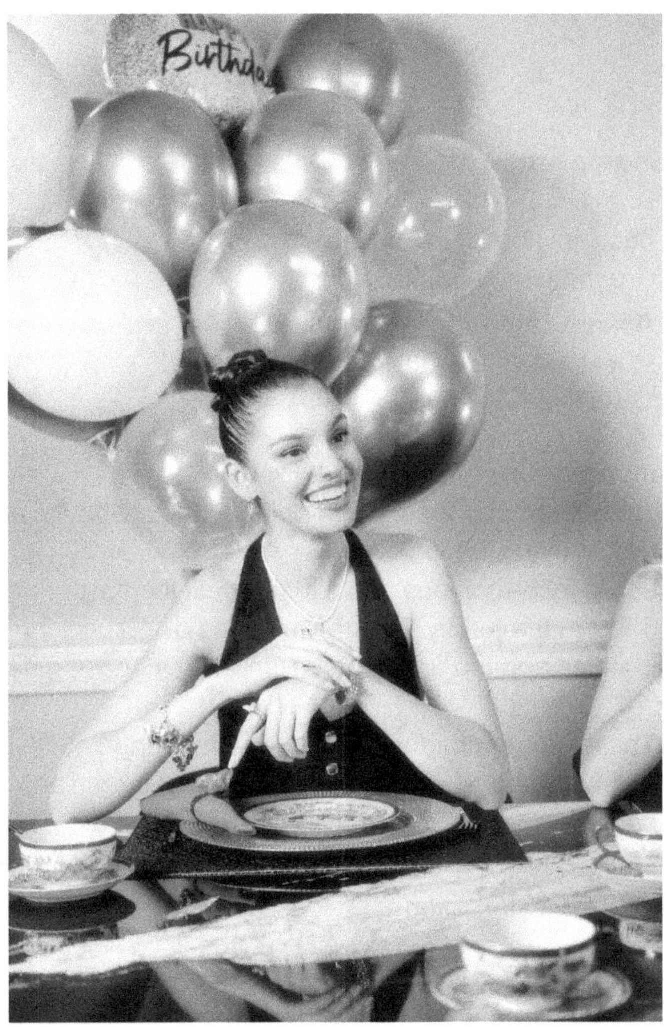

Instructions:
Season salmon with lemon zest, olive oil, and herbs if
desired, then bake or grill until cooked through.
Serve the salmon over a bed of cooked quinoa and
steamed greens.

Zucchini Noodles with Turkey Bolognese

Ingredients:

Zucchini noodles (zoodles)
Ground turkey or chicken
Tomato sauce (low sugar or homemade)
Onion, garlic, Italian herbs
Parmesan cheese (optional)

Instructions:
1.Sauté ground turkey with onions, garlic, and Italian herbs until browned.
2.Add tomato sauce and simmer until the flavours meld.
3.Serve the turkey Bolognese sauce over zucchini noodles and top with grated Parmesan cheese if desired.

These dinner creations offer a diverse range of flavours and nutrients while incorporating low GI ingredients to help maintain stable blood sugar levels. Adjust seasonings and ingredients according to personal taste preferences!

Delicious and easy-to-prepare low GI dinners for various tastes and preferences.

Absolutely! Here are some delicious and easy-to-prepare low glycemic index (GI) dinners that cater to various tastes and preferences:

Stuffed Bell Peppers

Ingredients:

Bell peppers (any colour)
Lean ground turkey or chicken
Quinoa or brown rice
Diced tomatoes, onions, garlic
Italian seasoning, salt, pepper
Low-sugar tomato sauce

Instructions:
1.Preheat oven to 375°F (190°C).
2 Cut the tops off bell peppers, remove seeds, and parboil for a few minutes.
3.In a skillet, sauté onions and garlic, then add ground turkey or chicken and cook until browned.
4.Add cooked quinoa or brown rice, diced tomatoes, Italian seasoning, salt, and pepper. Mix well.
5.Stuff the bell peppers with the mixture, place in a baking dish, pour tomato sauce over the peppers, and bake for 25-30 minutes until peppers are tender.

Lemon Garlic Herb Baked Salmon

Ingredients:
Salmon fillets
Lemon juice, minced garlic, fresh herbs (such as dill, parsley)
Olive oil, salt, pepper

Instructions:
1.Preheat oven to 400°F (200°C).

2.Mix lemon juice, minced garlic, fresh herbs, olive oil, salt, and pepper in a bowl.
3.Place salmon fillets on a baking sheet, brush with the prepared mixture.
4.Bake for about 12-15 minutes until the salmon is cooked through and flakes easily with a fork.

Mushroom and Spinach Quiche

Ingredients:
Whole grain pie crust or crustless option
Eggs, egg whites
Sautéed mushrooms, spinach, onions, garlic
Low-fat cheese (optional)
Salt, pepper, herbs

Instructions:
1.Preheat the oven to 375°F (190°C).
2.Line a pie dish with the whole grain pie crust or use a crustless option.
3.Whisk together eggs, egg whites, salt, pepper, and herbs.
4.Layer sautéed mushrooms, spinach, onions, garlic, and low-fat cheese in the pie crust.
5.Pour the egg mixture over the fillings and bake for 30-35 minutes until set.

Tofu Stir-Fry with Vegetables

Ingredients:

Firm tofu

Assorted vegetables (bell peppers, broccoli, carrots, snap peas)
Low-sodium soy sauce, garlic, ginger
Olive oil or sesame oil

Instructions:
1.Press tofu to remove excess water, then cut into cubes.
2.Stir-fry tofu in a pan with olive oil or sesame oil until lightly browned.
3.Add assorted vegetables, minced garlic, and ginger. Cook until vegetables are tender-crisp.
4.Stir in low-sodium soy sauce for flavour and serve.

These dinners are simple to prepare, packed with flavour, and cater to different tastes while adhering to a low GI lifestyle. Adjust ingredients and seasonings according to personal preferences!

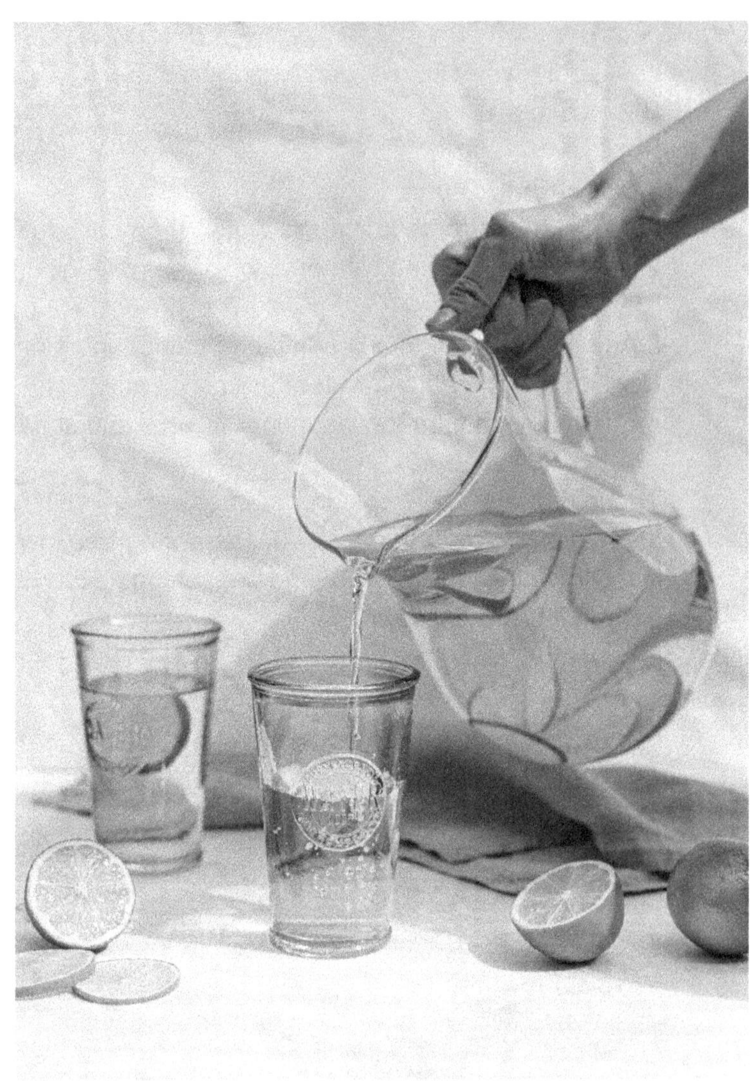

Chapter Seven

Smart Snacking Solutions

Absolutely! Smart snacking while following a low glycemic index (GI) diet involves choosing nutrient-dense options that help maintain stable blood sugar levels. Here are some ideas:

Nuts and Seeds

Almonds, Walnuts, and Pistachios:
These nuts are rich in healthy fats, protein, and fibre, making them a satisfying and low GI snack.

Chia Seeds, Flaxseeds: Packed with omega-3 fatty acids and fibre, these seeds can be added to yoghurt, smoothies, or homemade energy balls for a nutritious boost.

Greek Yoghourt with Berries
Plain Greek Yoghurt: High in protein and probiotics, choose unsweetened varieties.

Berries (Strawberries, Blueberries): Low GI fruits that add sweetness and antioxidants to your snack.

Hummus and Veggies

Chopped Vegetables (Carrots, Cucumber, Bell Peppers): Crunchy and low GI, perfect for dipping.
Hummus: A delicious dip made from chickpeas, offering protein and fibre.

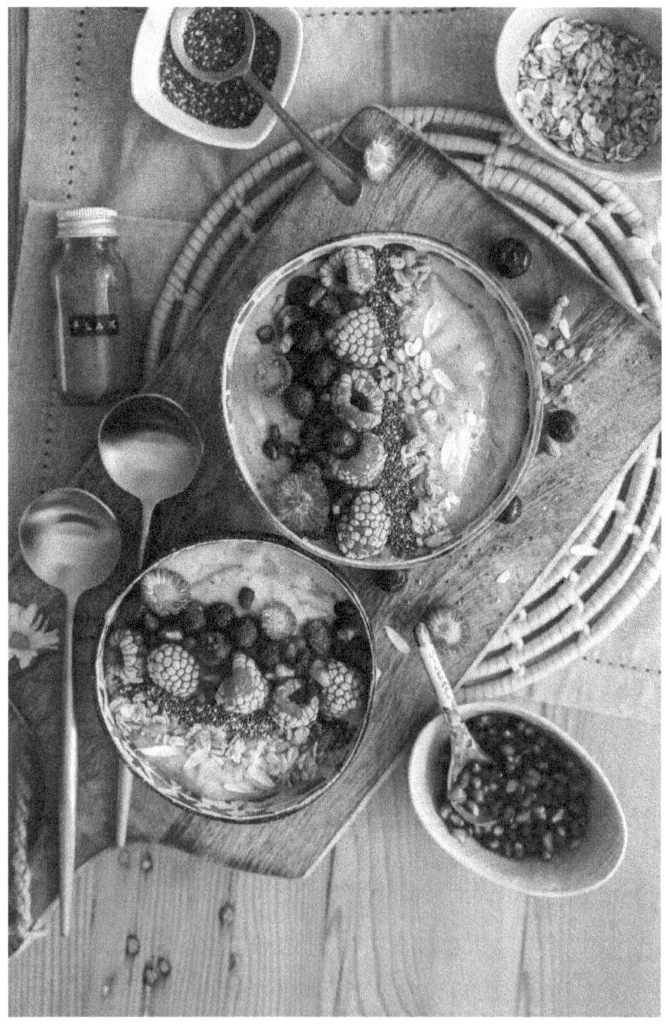

Hard-Boiled Eggs
Eggs: An excellent source of protein and various nutrients, easy to prepare in advance for on-the-go snacking.

Avocado on Whole Grain Crackers

Avocado: Rich in healthy fats and fibre, spread on whole grain crackers for a satisfying snack.

Homemade Trail Mix

Mix of Nuts, Seeds, and Dried Fruits: Create your own trail mix with almonds, pumpkin seeds, and dried apricots or cranberries for a balanced snack.
Vegetable Sticks with Guacamole or Salsa
Celery, Cucumber, and Carrot Sticks: Low GI options that pair well with guacamole or salsa for added flavour.

Edamame

Steamed Edamame: These young soybeans are a good source of protein and fibre, perfect for a nutritious snack.

Apple Slices with Peanut Butter

Apples: Choose varieties like Granny Smith, which have a lower GI.
Natural Peanut Butter: Opt for varieties with no added sugars for a satisfying dip.

Popcorn

Air-Popped Popcorn: A whole grain snack when prepared without excessive butter or sugary toppings.

Cottage Cheese with Pineapple

Low-Fat Cottage Cheese: High in protein and low in carbohydrates.
Pineapple: A sweet fruit option with a moderate GI when consumed in moderation.

Energy Bars or Protein Balls
Homemade or Low Sugar Options: Look for bars or balls made with whole ingredients and low in added sugars.

These smart snacking solutions offer a balance of nutrients, helping to curb hunger while keeping blood sugar levels steady throughout the day. Adjust portion sizes according to individual nutritional needs!

Healthy and low glycemic snack ideas to keep energy levels steady throughout the day.

1.Cottage Cheese with Berries
Low-fat Cottage Cheese: High in protein and calcium.
Berries (Strawberries, Blueberries): Low GI fruits rich in antioxidants.

2. Veggie Sticks with Hummus

Carrot, Celery, and Bell Pepper Sticks: Crunchy and low GI.
Hummus: A flavorful dip made from chickpeas, offering protein and fibre.

3. Hard-Boiled Eggs with Whole Grain Crackers
Hard-Boiled Eggs: A great source of protein and various nutrients.
Whole Grain Crackers: Choose crackers made from whole grains for added fibre.

4. Greek Yogurtparfait
Plain Greek Yoghurt: High in protein and probiotics.
Mixed Berries and a Sprinkle of **Nuts or Seeds**: Adds antioxidants and healthy fats.

5. Almonds and Dried Apricots
Almonds: Rich in healthy fats, protein, and fibre.
Dried Apricots: A sweet and low GI dried fruit option.

6. Rice Cakes with Avocado
Brown Rice Cakes: Low GI and a good source of whole grains.
Avocado Slices: Rich in healthy fats and fibre.

7. Tuna or Salmon Salad on Cucumber Slices
Canned Tuna or Salmon: High in protein and omega-3 fatty acids.
Cucumber Slices: Low GI and refreshing.

8. Edamame

Steamed Edamame: A plant-based protein snack with fibre.

9. Apple Slices with Nut Butter

Apple Slices: Choose varieties like Granny Smith for a lower GI.
Natural Nut Butter: Peanut, almond, or cashew butter for a satisfying dip.

10. Popcorn with Herbs

Air-Popped Popcorn: A whole grain snack when prepared without excessive butter or sugary toppings.
Herbs (like rosemary or thyme): Add flavour without extra calories.

11. Chia Seed Pudding

Chia Seeds soaked in Unsweetened Almond Milk: Rich in fibre and omega-3 fatty acids.
Topped with Berries or a Sprinkle of Nuts: Adds antioxidants and nutrients.

12. Mixed Nuts and Seeds

A Variety of Nuts (Almonds, Walnuts) and Seeds (Pumpkin, Sunflower): A satisfying mix of healthy fats and protein.
These snacks offer a blend of protein, healthy fats, and fibre to help stabilise blood sugar levels and provide lasting energy throughout the day. Incorporate them into your routine for a nutritious and satisfying snack time! Adjust portion sizes based on individual needs and preferences.

Chapter Eight

Desserts with a Low GI Twist

1.Berry Chia Seed Pudding: Combine chia seeds with unsweetened almond milk, a touch of vanilla extract, and fresh berries. Let it sit overnight for a delightful, naturally sweet pudding.

2.Sugar-Free Fruit Sorbet: Blend frozen fruits like berries, mango, or pineapple with a splash of coconut water or a bit of Greek yoghourt for a refreshing, naturally sweet sorbet.

3.Almond Flour-based Treats: Try baking with almond flour to create goodies like almond flour cookies, muffins, or cakes. They're lower in carbs and higher in protein compared to traditional flour-based desserts.

4.Yogurt Parfait with Berries: Layer Greek yoghourt with fresh berries, a sprinkle of nuts or seeds, and a drizzle of honey or a touch of stevia for a delightful, low-GI dessert option.

These desserts offer sweetness without the sugar spike, making them perfect for those following a low-GI diet.

Indulgent yet healthy dessert recipes that align with a low glycemic index diet.

Absolutely! Here are some indulgent yet healthy dessert recipes that align with a low glycemic index diet:

Dark Chocolate Avocado Mousse:

Blend ripe avocados, unsweetened cocoa powder, a touch of honey or maple syrup, and a splash of almond milk until smooth and creamy. Chill and serve for a rich, satisfying chocolate dessert.

Baked Apples with Cinnamon and Walnuts:

Core apples and fill the centres with a mix of chopped walnuts, cinnamon, and a hint of honey. Bake until tender for a warm, naturally sweet treat.

Coconut Flour Brownies:

Use coconut flour, unsweetened cocoa powder, eggs, a natural sweetener like stevia or monk fruit, and a bit of coconut oil to create fudgy, low-GI brownies that are both decadent and guilt-free.

Greek Yogurt Cheesecake with Nut Crust:

Make a cheesecake using Greek yoghourt, cream cheese, a nut-based crust (almond or walnut), and a natural sweetener. Bake it to perfection for a creamy, indulgent dessert.

These recipes offer the richness and satisfaction of classic indulgent desserts but with a mindful selection of ingredients that keep the glycemic index low, ensuring they fit well within a low-GI diet.

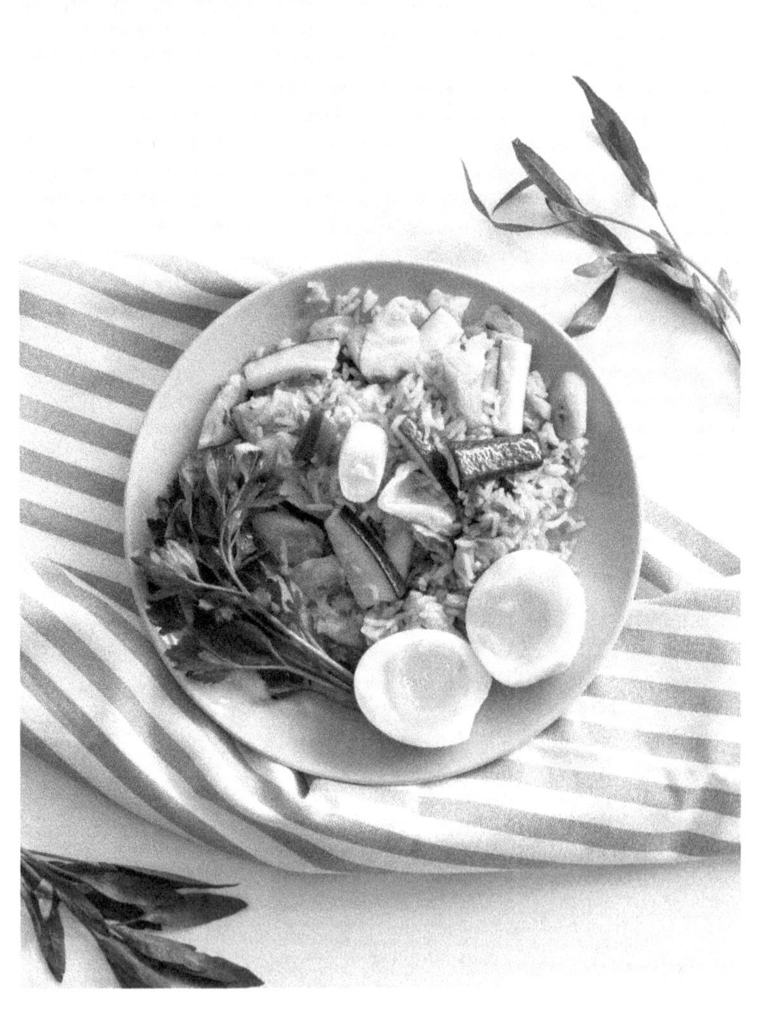

Chapter Nine

Sustaining Your Low GI Lifestyle

Maintaining a low glycemic index (GI) lifestyle is about more than just food choices; it's a holistic approach to wellness. Here's how to sustain it:

1.Balanced Meals: Focus on balanced meals combining lean proteins, healthy fats, and high-fibre carbohydrates. This balance helps regulate blood sugar levels and keeps you feeling full longer.

2.Mindful Eating: Pay attention to portion sizes and listen to your body's hunger cues. Slow down during meals, savour flavours, and avoid distractions to prevent overeating.

3.Regular Exercise: Incorporate regular physical activity into your routine. Exercise helps improve insulin sensitivity, managing blood sugar levels more effectively.

4.Stress Management: High stress can impact blood sugar. Practice stress-relieving activities like meditation, yoga, or hobbies to keep stress levels in check.

5.Hydration: Drink plenty of water throughout the day. Staying hydrated supports overall health and can aid in controlling hunger and cravings.

6.Meal Planning: Plan meals ahead to ensure you have low-GI options readily available. This reduces the temptation of reaching for high-GI foods when rushed or hungry.

7.Education & Awareness: Stay informed about the GI values of various foods. Knowledge empowers better food choices and helps you navigate dining out or grocery shopping with ease.

By incorporating these practices into your daily routine, you can sustain a low-GI lifestyle, promoting better health and well-being in the long run.

Strategies, tips, and advice on maintaining and integrating the low GI diet into everyday life for long-term success.

Absolutely, maintaining and integrating a low glycemic index (GI) diet into everyday life for long-term success involves several strategies and tips:

1.Education and Awareness: Learn about the GI values of different foods. Focus on consuming low-GI foods like non-starchy vegetables, whole grains, lean proteins, and healthy fats.

2.Meal Planning and Preparation: Plan meals in advance, emphasising low-GI ingredients. This practice makes it easier to stick to the diet, especially during busy days. Batch cooking can also be helpful.

3.Healthy Swaps: Replace high-GI foods with lower-GI alternatives. For instance, opt for whole grains instead of refined grains, and choose sweet potatoes over white potatoes.

4.Balanced Meals: Aim for balanced meals that include protein, healthy fats, and fibre-rich carbohydrates. This combination helps regulate blood sugar levels and keeps you satiated.

5.Snack Smartly: Have low-GI snacks available, like nuts, seeds, Greek yoghourt, or sliced vegetables with hummus, to curb cravings and maintain stable energy levels between meals.

6.Mindful Eating: Practise mindful eating by slowing down, chewing food thoroughly, and paying attention to hunger and fullness cues. This habit aids in better digestion and prevents overeating.

7.Regular Monitoring: Check in with your progress regularly. Monitor how your body responds to different foods and adjust your diet accordingly.

8.Stay Hydrated: Drink an adequate amount of water daily. Sometimes thirst can be mistaken for hunger, leading to unnecessary snacking.

9.Physical Activity: Incorporate regular exercise into your routine. It helps manage blood sugar levels and contributes to overall health and well-being.

10.Support and Flexibility: Surround yourself with a supportive environment. Also, be flexible with yourself – occasional deviations from the diet are normal and shouldn't discourage long-term commitment.

Integrating these strategies into your daily life gradually can make adopting a low-GI diet more manageable and sustainable for long-term success.

Conclusion

In conclusion, embracing a low glycemic index (GI) diet isn't just about altering eating habits; it's a journey toward a healthier lifestyle. By understanding the impact of foods on blood sugar levels and making mindful choices, you've embarked on a path that prioritises well-being and balanced nutrition.

Remember, this journey is unique for everyone. It's about finding what works best for your body and creating sustainable habits that support your health goals. Whether it's managing weight, improving energy levels, or promoting overall wellness, the low-GI lifestyle offers a framework that encourages nutritious, satisfying, and delicious eating.

As you continue on this path, staying informed, planning meals, making mindful choices, and integrating physical activity will serve as pillars of your success. Embrace the journey with patience and flexibility, celebrating the small victories along the way.

Here's to your continued commitment to health, vitality, and a delicious life guided by the principles of the low-GI diet! Cheers to your well-being and the vibrant journey ahead.

Backend keywords

1. Low glycemic index diet cookbook for dummies
2. Low glycemic index diet cookbook for seniors
3. Joydays low glycemic cookie
4. Low glycemic index food guide
5. Low glycemic index food chart
6. Low glycemic index food guide chart 2023
7. Low glycemic index protein powder

9 798875 569913